T0198513

# Preserving Your Precious Pouch

By Sylvia Rebecca Morris-Mccalla

To order additional copies of this book, contact:
Xlibris
844-714-8691
www.Xlibris.com
Orders@Xlibris.com

ISBN: 978-1-6641-3776-9 (sc)
ISBN: 978-1-6641-3775-2 (e)

Print information available on the last page

Rev. date: 11/17/2020

Dear Reader,

Presented here is a new body of knowledge, as ridiculous as it may seem, please accept it as the reality of millions of women on a daily basis. This book is to bring awareness about the situation to everyone. For those who think the content of this book is substandard for publishing, remember our children are carrying a world of pornography in their bags every day.

# Introduction

Presented here is the untold tale of an unpreserved pouch. The tale is about the pouch of Douglas and its relation to the buttocks and gluteal muscles. The gluteals were made to be tight and firm so that they can support the urogenital organs of the pelvic cavity; but for a senseless reason a young girl will walk and shake her gluteals.

The act of walking and shaking is simple and easy to do, but it's an obstetrical and gynecological disaster.

There is not a single positive outcome from walking and shaking the gluteals. It's an expensive habit, and psychologically challenging because it's impossible for her to maintain a healthy sexual relationship. However, all is not lost, complete rehabilitation can be achieved.

# What is the pouch of Douglas?

Anatomist James Douglas 1675-1742 was credited for discovering the pouch of Douglas, it is part of the female human anatomy that is hardly known and very rarely spoken of. In modern medicine the pouch of Douglas is known as the recto-uterine pouch or the posterior cul-de-sac. It is situated on the posterior wall of the pelvis behind the uterus in the female human body.

During sexual intercourse the penis enters directly into the pouch of Douglas; where, there is an accumulation of three to five milliliters of secretion during and after the female cycle. This secretion lubricates the vagina and a vacuum suction motion is produced during intercourse while thrusting back and forth.

Here in the pouch of Douglas is the birthplace of sexual gratification, ecstasy, and a lingering state of euphoria. It is this experience which brings a man back to a woman, leaves the woman with a sense of power in their relationship and a feeling of security. The pouch of Douglas can also be predisposed to the diseases such as cancer lesions, endometriosis and ascites just like the other reproductive organs.

# Female Pelvis Showing the pouch of Douglas

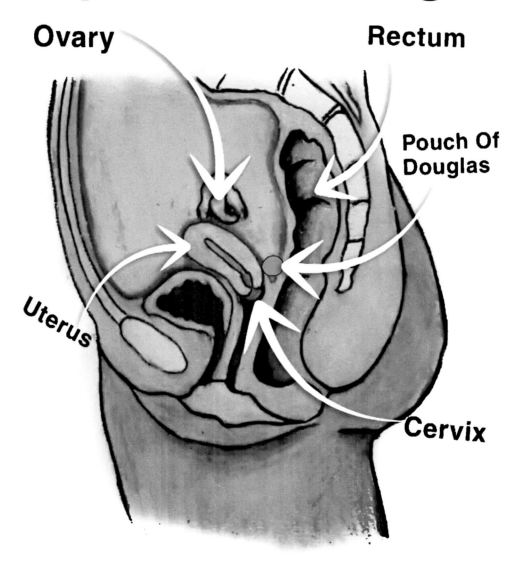

Ovary

Rectum

Pouch Of Douglas

Uterus

Cervix

# The Pelvic Basin

The pelvis in the human anatomy begins at the waist; it comprises of the ilium, ischium, sacrum, pubic bones, and the coccyx. Where the ilium meets the femur or thigh bones is called the hip. The pelvis joins the upper skeleton to the lower limbs and supports the spinal column. In addition to the bony structure, the pelvis also has a floor that is made of thick muscles as well as the three pairs of levator ani muscles that run laterally, anteriorly, and posteriorly. These muscles are thick, strong, and help to make up the pelvic basin; they also help prevent urine and fecal incontinence.

The coccygeus muscles originate from the ischium and joins the lateral aspect of the sacrum and the coccyx. The function of the pelvis is for walking and a general upright stance as well as providing protection for the urogenital organs and other abdominal organs.

# The Pelvic Basin

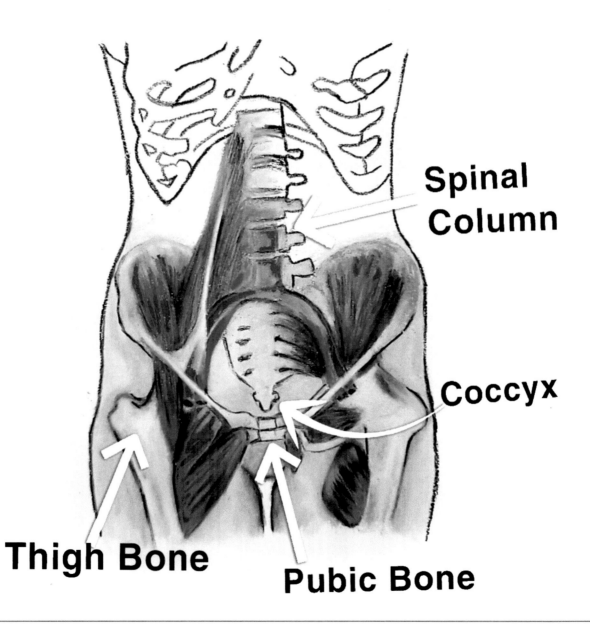

Spinal Column

Coccyx

Thigh Bone

Pubic Bone

# The Buttocks

The shape of the pelvis determines the shape of the buttocks; flat in most men and some women; and rounded in most females. The buttocks are situated in the back of the hip, has two cheeks, is formed by the joint of each thigh bone and the fleshy part of the upper thigh.

The buttocks are covered in the back by the gluteus maximus, the gluteus medius, and the gluteus minimus; they also protect the organs of the pelvic cavity. Nice firm gluteus and round pelvic bones underpin a nice firm buttock. It gives both a professional and a sexy look to any woman.

The buttock is the part of the woman's body that gets the most attention. It has the most nicknames, it is used as curse words, and the most jokes surround it. More than all the other structures of the human body, the buttocks attract the most compliments.

Men very often, describe a woman to their friends by how he sees her romp.

Having firm, sturdy, buttocks can only be accomplished with solid pelvic muscles and strong stable gluteal. With both groups of muscles intact, the urogenital organs are well protected and only then can the pouch of Douglas be felt. With strong solid muscles even when voiding a thrill can be felt.

Because of the strength of the supporting muscles and the pouch of Douglas lying sub-adjacent to the uterus; after a hysterectomy, the sexual experience remains the same as the penis goes exclusively into the pouch of Douglas.

Sciatica is the disorder associated with the buttocks in addition to other injuries.

# The Muscles In The Buttocks

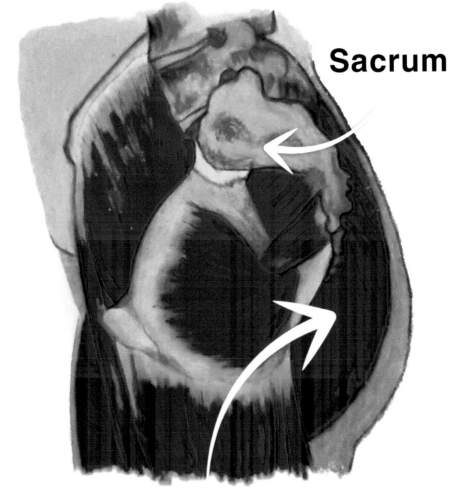

**Sacrum**

**Gluteus Maximus**

# The Opposite of a Sturdy Romp

A woman's esthetic and romp attract others to her. However, there is one factor that can negate her beauty it's the opposite of having nice sturdy gluteals. As a good firm buttock is a plus, and compliments are numerous. The opposite is experienced by every woman whose rear end has a rhythm of its own; whose gluteal are lax, limp, and flaccid.

The act of walking and shaking the gluteals has been always practiced by women of every race, nation, and socioeconomic standing. Yet this action has never been discussed at any level. The habit appears to be a simple act and a way of trying to be stylish, but it never looks stylish and after a while the opposite is attained. The consequences are horrendous and detrimental; it is far from being a simple act.

Walking itself is more difficult and the gait is unsteady. A woman who walks and shakes her gluteal is called derogatory names like "waterish pumpkin", "sappy arse", "bottom in the road", "muscle muscovado", and a vast number of other names. Walking and shaking the gluteal can easily be classified as one of the greatest acts of self-sabotaging one can commit. Maybe it's one of the few conditions where the perpetrator and the victim is the same person. Not even the victim herself can figure out what the problem is.

# To Whom Does She Go To?

A drug addict has family and friends in his or her pavilion encouraging him/her to get off drugs, but a woman who walks like that is lucky if one friend or family member will draw her attention to the issue. Even after she is told about the way she walks she feels powerless to reverse her action. Such a woman has a lonely existence and is suffering in silence.

Within her private circle of friends and family; her stock is so low and mistrust high. Without the slightest provocation her best friend will tell others "I am sure that "waterish pumpkin" is sleeping with my husband."

Statements like these will be dismissed or a sister will say, "Why are you always speaking to my husband, where is yours? You, slobbery arse!"

An even more unhealthy dose of mistrust is when a stranger says that she is a lesbian and everyone believes without any given evidence except for one statement, "He opened his mouth wide and talked!"

# Low Self-esteem

The female with flaccid gluteals is handicapped by low self-esteem. If she sees someone walking the way she does she might say to herself in disgust, "So that's how common I look!" She accepts the fact that her company of employment will never send her to a conference to represent them she perceives it's because of her rear end.

If two men approach her, asking to start a relationship, automatically she will choose the lesser developed of the two; because she believes he will be more accepting of her and the way she walks. She might say to herself, "They didn't invite me to appear at the fashion show because of this worthless behind I have!" the poor woman is plagued with hopelessness. She is ashamed to walk pass a group of men, or one of her rivals.

# The Female Pelvic Organs In Relation To The Other Organs

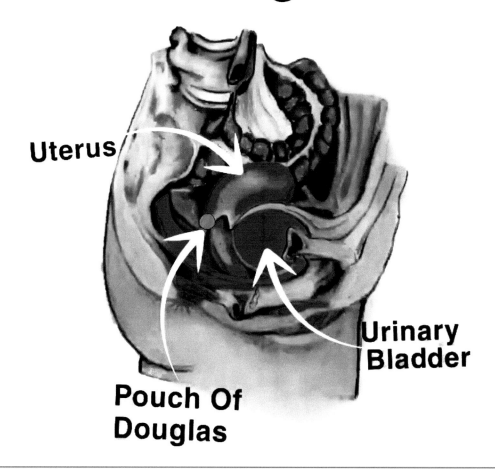

Uterus

Urinary Bladder

Pouch Of Douglas

# Effects on the Relationship

Even more devastating than the mental anguish, is her inability to maintain a healthy sexual relationship. She knows her husband is dissatisfied with her performance in bed, but all she has is an overwhelming feeling of being a failure.

The question often asked is, "I wonder where I'm going wrong?"

The matter is too personal for her to discuss with anyone. She knows her husband is cheating and wishes she was the other woman.

Other ways of expressing the disappointment is, "I'm not keeping a partner, as soon as he gets what he wants he is gone!" She knows that he doesn't want what he got so he never returned. She might say, "He wined and dined me for one year, all of a sudden he has stopped visiting!" But what was excluded from that statement is, "After one night in bed he never called or visited again!"

Every relationship is the last try because she still needs the support of a husband

A little girl who was never promiscuous and who was raised by a mother who can easily qualify for the title of the world's most stable woman; how can that same girl now be classified as a promiscuous woman?

# Wearing Restrictive Garments

Physically walking becomes a chore for her, so wearing a girdle is the option used to restrict the movements of the gluteals. But adding a tight girdle to muscles that are already limp and flabby, softens them further; this adds more stress to the pelvic organs that are already over stressed by the muscles that are supposed to protect them.

When her peers are wearing G-strings, bikini swimsuits, and other flimsy underwear she has to invest in expensive girdles and restrictive under garments.

A Dentist exams his client and sees his/her teeth are growing out of alignment and recommend braces to him/her. Yet women who have been walking that way for generations an obstetrician or gynecologist has never made the connection between walking, shaking the gluteal and a woman's reproductive health.

With the constant bombardment caused by over activity of the muscles of the pelvic floor it loses its elasticity, the uterus is often lying lower in the pelvis than is normal. The pouch of Douglas is non-existent, and the cervix is now lying in front of it.

Therefore, the cervix is bombarded during intimacy, in a normal situation the penis should never touch the cervix.

With the pouch of Douglas gone the secretions that it produces and acts as a lubricant during intercourse is now in the vagina, so she is always in a state of wetness.

Lax pelvic muscles increased vaginal secretions and a cervix lower in place than it should be is not a good recipe for an enjoyable sex life neither for healthy reproductive organs. The cervix is in a constant state of wetness and is predisposed to tearing during labor and delivery. A torn cervix predisposes a woman to cervical cancer.

# Female Pelvis

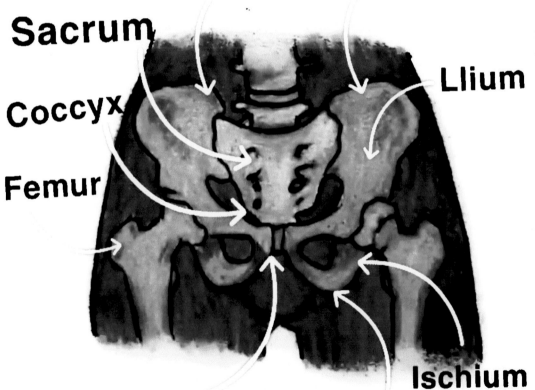

Sacroiliac spine

Lliac Crest

Sacrum

Llium

Coccyx

Femur

Ischium

Pubic Symphysis

Pubic Bone

# One Size Fits All

Australian Tracy Sorensen said the pouch of Douglas is a piece of nothing.

Sorry Stacy I beg to differ, and I'd like to prove you wrong scientifically at a later date.

There is not one accomplishment to achieve by walking and shaking one's romp. Yet, fat and thin women, poor and rich women, short and tall women, who walk and shake their romps have become victims of their own choice.

A subdeb who walks and shakes her romp will go through life without experiencing the pleasure and satisfying life that a sound pouch of Douglas affords.

Instead she will forever live under a cloud of suspicion of infidelity, and queries about the paternity of her children. She is most likely to end up single.

# Another Reason for Preserving Your Precious Pouch

Every religion emphasizes the importance of the sacredness of the human body.

Christianity depends on it.

"Therefore, shall a man leave his father and mother, and shall cleave unto his wife and the two shall become one flesh." Genesis 2:24.

This world is plagued with the ill effects of premarital sex, yet it is treated like a special commodity, and the woman who remains chaste until marriage is called stupid.

Sex is the only action a man and a woman doesn't have to practice ensuring a successful relationship.

Romans 12:1 "Says I beseech you therefore, brethren by the mercies of God that ye present your bodies a living sacrifice, holy, acceptable unto God which is your reasonable service."

Every young woman is encouraged to preserve her precious pouch and exchange it only for love and a stable relationship.

# The Muscles In The Pelvis

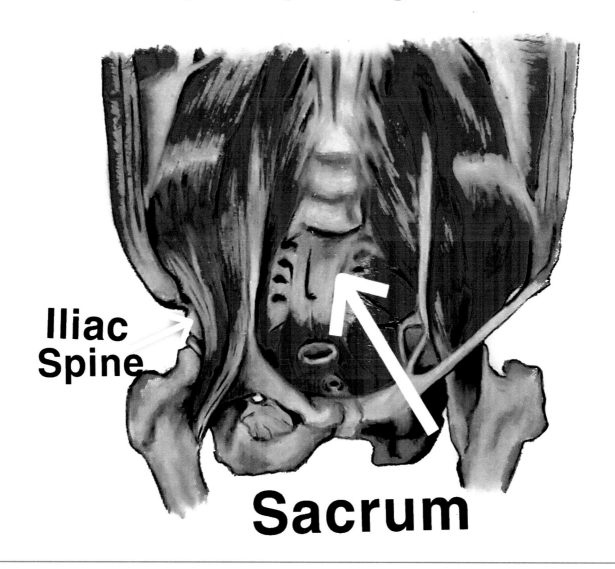

Iliac Spine

Sacrum

# The Survey

The information presented here was not scientifically tested neither was it pulled out of a hat; but was compiled by a group of women who took part in a survey. This information was gleaned from their previous experiences and not only from their subjectivity.

Twelve women participated in the survey, seven of the twelve were never married and had children for several fathers. Three were married and are now divorced, they remained single. Of the other two, their husbands are having extramarital relationships and extramarital children.

However, the group had to agree that there are many women who walk poised and lady-like, yet their husbands are unfaithful, so this information will be useful to them as well. It was also observed by the participants that men don't walk shaking their gluteal muscles; perhaps doing that is a personal choice because among the group only three participants knew a total of three men walking that way. **There are no visible** elderly women walking that way.

Muscles have memory, rehabilitation can be complete, and everyone will benefit from doing some exercises for the gluteus.

They weren't able to determine the effects of twerking on the gluteus.

# Bringing About an Awareness

The group consensus was that rehabilitation of gluteal muscles can be simple, swift, and effective.

The first step to rehabilitation must be to bring an awareness of this nameless condition, which is walking and shaking the gluteals; by both(a) the victims and (b)by professional and those in authority.

The expectations are this booklet will enlighten the initial step towards bringing about an awareness; that the new body of knowledge presented here will be accepted and promoted by those in authority.

Ultimately others might not perceive it as joke or mockery but will be supportive of those women who need their support.

# The New Exercise

Every exercise will help; however, a new exercise was created to match the new form of rehabilitation. It was named "Bouncy-Bounce" all that is needed is a pair of tennis shoes and a sturdy surface such as a kitchen sink to hold on to. The method is simply hold on to the sink with both hands, lean forward, extend the rear end, legs apart, and bounce on the soles of your feet. The idea is to engage or tighten the entire pelvic and gluteal muscles.

Complete rehabilitation can be accomplished after thirty days, one hour per day
(The expectation is this exercise will be tested to rule out th possibility of injury to surrounding joints and tissues)

Other forms of exercise such as walking, stair climbing, Kegel maneuver, weight training, resistance band exercises, Goblet squats are necessary in maintaining the gluteals after the initial rehabilitation.

# A Normal Life

The effect of years of feeling downtrodden will come to an end and wearing tight girdles will be a habit of the past. Choosing a date from the bottom of the pile will no longer be necessary. A whole new era will be ushered in with improved muscularity of the pelvic floor, the gluteus muscles, and a restored pouch of Douglas.

As a result, one's self confidence and assertion will be evident. One's date or companion will suggest you reveal your bottom by lifting your shirt above your waist. Your partner might say, "I haven't eaten for the day I'm still cherishing what you gave me last night."

"I couldn't imagine it was that good, take A plus!"

Out of jealousy a girlfriend might say, "Do you expect he will marry you, sorry he only wants you for what he can get from you!"

At last a man wants what is there to offer. Thanks to rehabilitation!

**Brett Jones, Ms. ATC CSCS** said, "walking, running, jumping, changing direction, and just about everything is better with strong gluteus." But he didn't mention sex; so, sex will be added. sex is better with good strong gluteal or sex is only good with firm solid gluteal.

# The Conclusion

Now that the tale of the restored pouch of Douglas has been told, it is hoped women the world over will consider the significance of the information attained here and implement it in their daily lives. In addition, those in authority will take this observation seriously and give credence for further study.

# Glossary

Arse: The buttocks

Muscovado: poor quality

Muscolosity: Muscle strength

Subdeb: A young girl just starting life

Sub-adjacent: Immediately below

*So, I'll highlight my darkest scene in ink of gold and green*
*Then I'll leave my book wide open for all the world to read."*
**The end**

# One Single Lover

I'm just asking for one single lover
One lover, one hand to hold,
Same dirty laundry to unfold
Those same pair of lips to kiss
and same pair of shoulders to cry on

At nights when I lay me down, I'll know what
to expect when I look around
One key to shut and lock life's door,
same tricky thoughts to decode
When the perfume is overnight and stale,
there'll be the same odor to inhale

When offsprings come along,
let them all be one
Same bad temper to control,
same facial features to behold
It's the only time when one is more
This sharing up is just not for me,
one single lover it would be

Young ones, stop and listen to this plea,
this sharing up just shouldn't be
I know you will agree with me,
one single lover let it be.
And when you are old and weary

and all you have left are memories
I know they will be good and bad,
let those memories be made with one.
So let me have just one single lover

# Other poems

# A Friend So True

I will thank the Master for a friend so true
Your compassionate and caring ways
You listen to my secret fears
You are my best example of what true friends can do

I would like to thank the Master for a friend in you
For the way you helped me bear my burdens
When I had no one to turn to
You are a strong tower through the torrents of my life

I would like to thank the master for a friend in you
When I was in need, you cooked the meal and spread the table
You are my strong haven
When my tides were heading towards the sea

I would like to thank the master that you are still around
One day I'll take my turn
To be a friend indeed
Master, thank you for my friend

# Calypso Sermon

Mama these little ones are under pressure
There is marijuana in every corner
Every morning you wake up there is a new murder
The world is setting them up for failure
When I think of their inheritance, I can see the war in Afghanistan
and the beach without sand
We asked them to have one safe sex partner,
yet right in the house they are distressed by their fathers
What is their inheritance? AIDS—Aids

Mama dress them up in what they have
these children know no pride
Walk down the road the first church you meet walk right in
the doors are open wide
Introduce them to the Pastor, Mama
Then take them every day they will grow brave and strong
Yet childlike in behavior

# Dear Jay,

I will ever bless the day you walked into my life
Your bravery is the center of my thoughts
You left your world behind to find me
You walked past scores of younger,
Beautiful, women who think they are more deserving of you.
You are my first and only experience of true love

I never knew a soft place to fall until you came through
my door
How nice it is to know someone who can see the interior
of my heart
Someone whose soul can keep company with mine
Just the sound of your voice makes me feel secure
Your comforting touch relaxes me even more
Please don't ever change, I love you just the way you are
You are really my only experience of true love
You have already won my heart.

# Dedicated to the family of the late Carlie Brucia and all other families who suffered the same loss.

*Rosebud so tender so sweet*
*From the seed you came almost complete*
*We watched over you and watered your roots*
*Waiting for you to open was our sacred treat*

In the garden of life you budded alright
*Your petals still folded*
*Your color so light*
*Of our beautiful rose we have now lost sight*

*The thorns and thistles surround you so fierce*
*Your beauty and splendor they have now laid waste*

*In the Garden of Eden we hope you bloom*
*Where bees can spread your pollen and your nectar consume*

*Carlie Carlie [s] rosebud so white*
*Life is so cruel and quite often no t right*
*Rosebud so strong yet so bright*
*We miss you, we miss you and this is our plight..*

## *Heaven's child*

Today, I thank the heaven for a child like you
Sometimes I wonder what I've done to deserve a gift so true
Your charisma and your politeness are the highlights of my life
So I thank heaven for its child

Again I will like to thank the heaven for a child
Who reminds me how to pray, and reads the word every day
Sometimes when you smile at me, I remember God's command
Thank heaven for a child like you

The serious way you tread life's path
The things that you have learnt
Reminds me how I live and love
You are a gift to a mother's heart

Sometimes I pull the curtain just to catch a glimpse of you
The simple way you plant your steps
Reminds me to be true
I thank God for heaven's child that's you.

# If the Moon can remember

If the moon can remember,
When you took me from my mother
Oh so pure and tender, I was never touched by another
If only the moon can remember.

I bore your child with dignity, amidst mountains of adversity
And the way it hurt my family
You said one day you will marry me
If only the moon can remember.

The moon was waning, my heart paining
You said youth is folly and love can't see
So with speed you changed your loyalty
You were really too blind to see

Now your heart is homeless and you are running wild
Your sister keeps complaining to my only child
Again I'm the one to listen to the tale of woes
While I'm still remembering the moonlight long ago

Chorus
You looked so lovely in the moon that shone
When you promised you'll be mine alone


_____,_____

(someone's name) (name repeated)
Why should it be a dream

_____

# I'm Free

Though I was born in sin and shaped in iniquity, your redeeming love has found me
Now my soul is free

How long did sin try to separate me from your pardoning grace and mercy
But your redeeming blood has bought me, now my soul is free

Now my name is written in the
Lamb's Book of Life
All because your redeeming love has found me, thank God my soul is free

I'm free, I'm free, thank God I'm free, thank God I'm free
I was born in sin and shaped in iniquity but
My name is now written in the Lamb's Book of Life
I'm free, I'm free, thank God I'm free

# Lonely Love Child

I thought my life was perfect and in line
and my Daddy's love sublime
Until I discovered I'm my father's outside child
My father's wife is furious, Mom invaded her private space
How could she do better when she's asked to share love
No woman wants another breathing in her husbands face.

My siblings are off limits, they call me" Daddy's bastard child"
I know they can't think otherwise, when their happiness is at stake
I who was a precious love child is now an appendage to a family
Oh how I wish my father was a carpenter, even though he couldn't see.

# Pearl of Precious Price

You started out so promising, your future looked so bright
We tried our best to teach you that childhood was a stride.

You keep shopping for your lovers
Your scruples are so loose
We thought you will wait to be discovered
and be someone's pearl of precious price

We could hardly recognize you
The way you wear your hair
Your clothes are so revealing
Your skin is almost bare

Sometimes at nights we howl
To see what you have learnt
The way you hop from bed to bed
And the places you enjoy

Chorus: Is she our pearl or is she that little girl
Please please remember she is still our
Precious pearl and not that little girl

# Rahab and the scarlet thread

When I think of the scarlet thread
I remember Rahab's faith
Not only the faith that comes from hearing
But the one from doing too

How her faith in God was grounded
Just to hear of the dried red sea
How the hearts did melt
To hear of the two kings Sihon and Og

By faith she recognized the spies
And the Lord who sent them too
She uttered words of courage
And obeyed what she ought to do

The line of scarlet thread bound in her window
She used to save the spies
That was her faith in action
As her father's house was next in line

Lord, my scarlet thread hangs in my window
Now give me Rahab's faith
So that I will salvation find
Then give me yet more faith
So that my family will be next in line

# The Little Girl And The Queen

Little girl little girl where have you been?
I went to Peruvian Vale to get a glimpse of the Queen
Little girl little girl what did you wear?
My old school clothes tattered and my feet bare
Little girl little girl what did you get there?
I saw the Queen wave while me alone cheered

Isn't it nice to see the Queen twice?
Once when you are eleven,
And then when you are thirty- seven.

I knew she wouldn't recognize me
Although I had taken another long journey
This time to England's West Minister Abbey
Highly seated in the front row across from the Queen
,by this I knew that I had grown-up
As I was so well dressed up in high heeled boots and make-up

Yes it is nice to see the Queen twice

# The Towers Three

This is the story of three towers no one two and three
The first was Babel in Babylon it stood
The children of men built it and they wouldn't be restrained
Until their language was confounded and they were scattered
all around

Next was Siloam tower it represented human strength and dignity
But it came tumbling and slew the eighteen who were scrambling
In Jerusalem the question was asked were they worst sinners
than all who dwelt here?

Third place went to the sisters—twin one and two
They stood in New York City brave and proud
Until one day they were turned upon

In the good old book the tale is written of towers one and two
Where would the tale of the sisters be written?
Who would tell the tale? who would ask the question
And what will the answer be?
Were they worst men than all others dwelling on earth?

Printed in the United States
By Bookmasters